CONTENTS

PREFACE

An old man is twice a child.

Hamlet, Act II, Scene ii, 391 **Shakespeare**
(Often quoted by Catfish as an old Scottish proverb.)

This monograph is based on a personal encounter with one of the notable herbalists of the Appalachian mountains, Clarence Frederick Gray, also known as 'Mr. Catfish Man of the woods'.

Mr. Catfish lived in a one room cabin on the banks of the Ohio River near Glenwood in Mason County. Anyone who had the opportunity to meet him was impressed by his humble and frank manners. He had genuine desire to help others who asked his opinion regarding herbal medicines.

He voluntarily met people from early morning until late evening, without taking a break. Due to his large herb garden in his backyard, I had the opportunity to examine more herbs than I had previously examined in the National Herb Garden in Washington D.C. He was a born naturalist with a keen eye to the observation and study of nature.

He remained very skeptical of modern medicine men and deeply felt that modern medical doctors are dishonest and greedy. This mutual suspicion of herbalist and medical doctors was quite obvious during our discussion. Mr. Catfish's mistrust in the medical profession was not much different from an old Roman saying:

"Until recently Dianulus was a doctor, now he is an undertaker. He is still doing as an undertaker what he used to do as a doctor."
---Martial Eigram

I last visited Mr. Catfish around Christmas 2001. He appeared fatigued and ill. Despite his healthy life style and love of nature, he was not able to escape Time's scythe.

When I do count the clock that tells the time,

And see the brave day sunk in hideous night;

...

Since sweets and beauties do themselves forsake

And die as fast as they see other grow;

And nothing 'gainst Time's scythe can make

Defense. Save breed, to brave him when he takes

thee hence.

Sonnet, XII
Shakespeare

Following a brief illness later in the year, he had passed away and was buried in a nearby family cemetery.

LIFE ON THE

OHIO RIVER

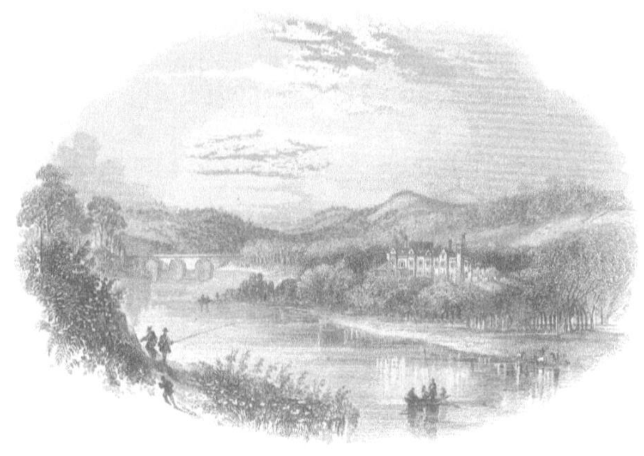

I concoct many lectuaries

that you may not find in any apothecaries.

You cannot beg any heart to whine apothecaries

let us start to commence to begin.

Canterbury Cat Tails
Hassan Amjad
Pilgrimage on River Ohio
With Apologies to
Geofrey

EARLY HISTORY OF CATFISH

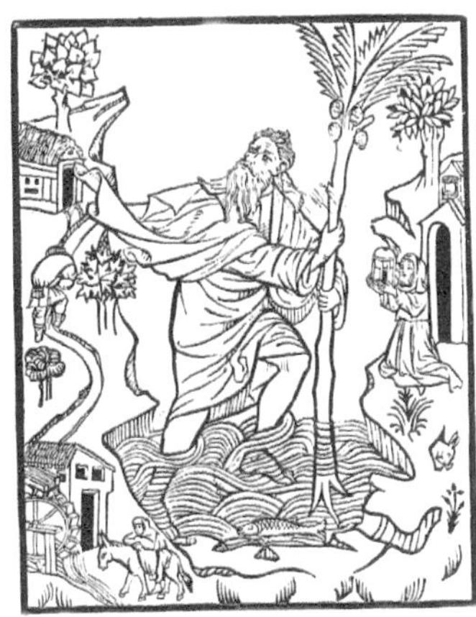

Mr. Clarence Frederick Gray was born on September 9th, 1917, on the Jackson and Roan County line, one mile from Liverpool West Virginia.[1] He recalled his ancestors back to the year 1870, when Arthur Seward Gray and Nancy Daurghty got married. He was a saw mill man and farmer. A boy was born 1874, named Boughrly Clayton Gray. He grew up and married at age 27 to 15 year old Della Dillon (who was the 13th child in the family of Abner Dillon, the year was 1907).

Clarence Frederick Gray married Mary Frances in 1942, both had 10 children.

---

1 Mr. Catfish was born in divided chicken coupe, 10 x 14 feet middle of the county line according to him he had a birth certificate from both counties.

"I am not as most people have, I was a poor boy most of my life, without any education and found my way in the dark to where I am now."

"Following God's finger as he pointed out the way for me to do."

"Its good to know that if you try once and can not succeed try try again. It is good as you wish just say it could have been worse, its good to know things half done is never done still."

--Mr. Catfish

Mr. Clarence Frederick Gray spent a great amount of time with his granddad Dillon near Sandyville, West Virginia. He taught him about herbs, a knowledge he had received from the Indians in 1861.

Many personal details of Mr. Catfish are not mentioned here at his request and a complete copy of his "Papyrus Catfishii" is at the Herb Academy. Knowledge of herbs came to his great-great grandfather who was taught by a Cherokee medicine man. He lived in several locations in West Virginia and Ohio, but always near the Ohio River. He gathered herbs around a small modest Cabin just outside Glenwood, in the area where Putnam, Mason, and Cabell counties converge.

For many years Mr. Catfish did not collect herbs, he worked at odd jobs to support his family. A fellow employee at DuPont Company gave him the name, '**Catfish**', during the time when he locally caught and sold catfish to workers at their quitting time. He injured both arms on a construction site and supported his family by selling wild flowers in Huntington.

Mr. Catfish always thought it was God's will to get in touch with nature and herbal medicine. While he was selling wildflowers, people started asking his opinion about treating different illnesses with herbs. Apparently in 1950 and 1960, Mr. Catfish developed some heart problems (I assume it was rheumatic heart disease) but he never believed in modern medicine, he remained a critic and skeptic.

> **"Living in harmony with nature assures a long, healthy life."**
>
> **--Mr. Catfish**

In my opinion, Mr. Catfish's thinking and philosophy of healing has a thread of common universal recurring themes. Whether it's Ayurvedic (science of life), Ancient Greek and Hippocratic Medicine also called Nature of Man's, Middle Eastern Sufis and mystic or Chinese philosophy of medicine. The basic underlying common thread is to fill these arts of healing by living in harmony with nature and with moderation to ecology, which may lead to a long life of happiness.

Regarding Mr., Catfish, perhaps the English Puritan preacher John Bunyan would have said: **A kind gentle Christian who spent his life well in caring of suffering of others, and will not seek self benefits, glory and honors.**

He Was A Devoted Christian

"I go to church twice a week, Sunday and Wednesday, and often as possible. I don't sell any of dope, liquor, wine or tobacco or marihuana, heroine or opium or any poisonous plants as nightshade, poison hemlocks, blue cohosh."

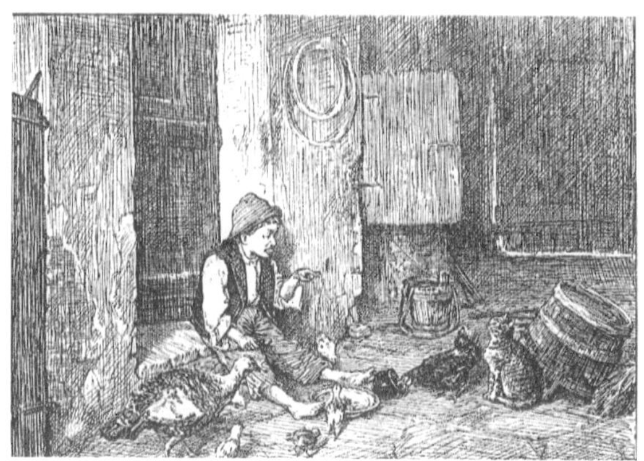

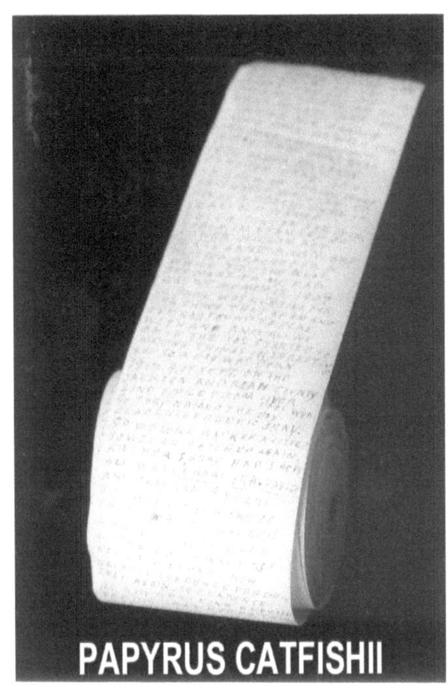

PAPYRUS CATFISHII

PAPYRUS CATFISHII

Many years ago, Mr. Catfish chose to write about himself, he took a large roll of Toledo Cash Register tape and started writing his autobiography. After many years past by, that roll of paper disappeared (it rolled under some furniture) but was found years later. He then had the opportunity to make a copy of it. Some of its contents which are relevant to him being an herbalist are present. Any detailed information about his personal life is NOT included.

A Work Routine for Catfish

12 sacks of Queen of Meddau

Set up his Herbs at home

7 sacks of Catnip

5lb Ginseng Dug.

4 BU. Golden Seal

Taught 2 more classes at Marshall

7 Bushel Slipper Elm

Talk at Public Library

Poison Ivy and Milk weed

MEDICAL ANTHROPOLOGY

OF

HERBS IN AMERICA

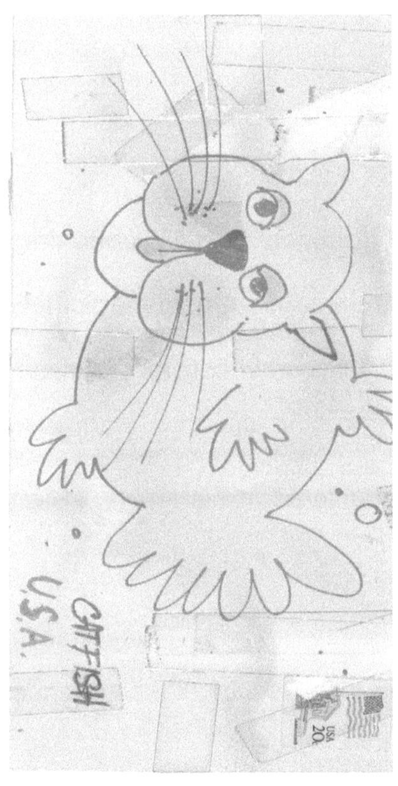

MR. CATFISH AND MEDICAL ANTHROPOLOGY OF HERBAL MEDICINE IN AMERICA

Over the years, Mr. Catfish received thousands of letters sent to him from various folks from surrounding states, and as far away as Florida, California, and even Europe. At one time, he had more than 50,000 letters, many of which were destroyed due to poor storage conditions. I had the opportunity to read several thousands of these letters. It allowed me a unique chance to look into the window of folk-herbal medicine in America.

I raised a simple question:

What are the common medical conditions for which people seek help outside conventional medicine?

Based on the communications of several thousand inquiries and myself reading hundreds of letters, I asked Mr. Catfish what are the common illnesses that he encountered in his letters. His responses are listed below:

They want treatment for:

1. Obesity – more than 50% of all letters requested some help, this was an early survey in 1980.
2. Arthritis and rheumatism
3. Something to improve sex life
4. Cancer (usually 3 or 4th most requested)

5. High Blood Pressure
6. Heart problems and diabetes
7. Warts
8. PMS, hot flashes

It also reflects, that one third of American's who are overweight, and hypertensive are the same population who suffers from arthritis, diabetes, and sexual problems! Herbal medicine, at least offers allure and promises of that "Elixir" or Alchemist's Pot of Gold. Does it deliver this promise it is itself a subject of a separate essay, at present the answer is a qualified: YES.

Herbal medicine is helpful in weight loss, arthritis, improving postmenopausal symptoms, and increasing libido. More people have asked Mr. Catfish's opinion about these health matters than any physician in the U.S. could ever dream of his entire life time.

CATFISH'S APOTHECARY

AND

GARDEN OF HERBS

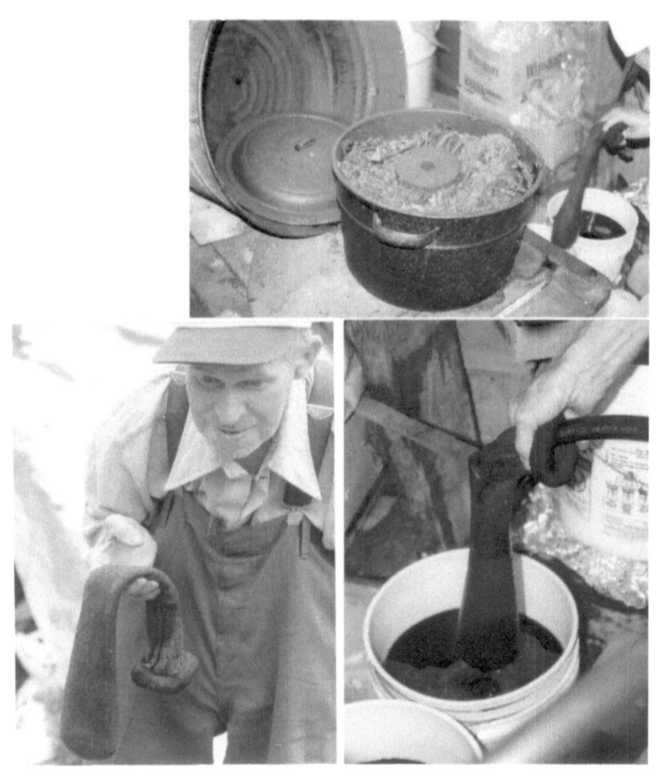

ALL HEALS THAT ENDS WELL

In my **garden of herbs** are stored

many things of sweet accord

Spices and sugar I combine

bitters and purges I divine

To strengthen the weak and sickly

Refreshing **sassafras teas** I furnish quickly

All these with utmost care

On all concoctions I prepare

--Hassan Amjad

With Apology to Hans Sachs

1568

WHEN AND HOW TO COLLECT HERBS

- Barks can be gathered in the spring or fall.
- Flowers should be gathered when the sun shines on them, as long as they retain their color and smell good.
- Seeds are good for many years.
- Roots are best when you dry them near a fire, and can last a long time.
- Leaves should be collected in clear, dry weather in the morning, and then they should be spread out thinly to dry.

GINSENG

Panax quinquefolium

A perennial herbaceous plant, flowers are greenish-yellow, with berries that are crimson-red. The roots have been used in Appalachia, kept in whiskey for days and used as a tonic. Despite the fact that West Virginia is the second highest producer of American Ginseng (after Kentucky), ginseng is still not popularly taken by West Virginians. However, many Chinese people value ginseng as an aphrodisiac.

Note: Ginseng is remarkably good **because it gives energy and decreases fatigue**, **the author recommends soaking** ginseng root overnight in water, which makes it swell up to a freshly dug state, which makes it easier to slice with a kitchen knife into small button size pieces. Take 1-2 pieces a day, slowly chewing; the maximum continuous use is 8-10 days. **Mr. Catfish** recommended **ginseng with ginger root** mixed together and used as a fine 'sex up tonic'.

MYRRH

Balsamodendron myrrha

It is known since ancient Biblical writings. The resin acts as an antiseptic, stimulant, tonic, and expectorant. It is useful for cough and asthma. If mixed with golden seal it is good for infections.

PLANTAIN

Plantago major

> **Romeo, Your plantain leaf is excellent for that**
>
> **Benvulvo for what I pray the Romeo for your**
>
> **Broken skin.**
>
> --Romeo and Juliet
> Shakespeare

A common flowering weed, leaves are bread flowery, with spikes of 3-5 inches. Fresh leaves can help heal cuts and bruises; it is also useful in the dressing of wounds.

RATS BANE (PIPSISSEWA)

Chimaphila Umbellata

It is a small herbaceous plant less than a foot tall with dark green leaves, which are toothed, and small reddish flowers. It is helpful for good urine flow and a good bitter tonic that helps fever. It is also good for kidney disease, infection of the lungs, and rheumatism. It was very highly valued by the Indians of Southern Appalachia.

BLACK CHERRY

Prunus serotina

Black cherry is a tall tree with dark bark, and leaves of 2-5 inches long. It has white flowers with round black cherries. A bark tea is useful for cough, colds, and to relieve muscle soreness. Black cherry was used to treat fever, intestinal worms, and to cure indigestion. The berries are dried and used to make a tea to help control diarrhea.

SUMACH BERRIES

Rhus glabra

The berries and stem bark have been combined with white pine and slippery elm, and have been used to treat syphilis. It has also been used for diabetes, fever, and sore throat.

SPIKENARD

Aralia racemosa

Spikenard is a perennial bush, with heart-shaped leaves like a canopy; it has greenish yellow flowers in clusters or a stalk. The root is medicinal. Tea made from the root is used for backache, treatment of chest colds, asthma, and increased sweating. It was used by Indians to shorten childbirth and was very popular.

COMFREY

Symphytum officinale

Comfrey has been known since ancient Greek times. It is useful to treat cough and internal kidney bleeding. A tea was made for external bruises, swelling and sprains, and it was also useful as poultice for skin boils. The effect of hot tea applied to bruises and sprains is due to the presence of allatoin, a chemical which promotes healing. Recent studies show it contains alkaloids which can cause liver damage and cancer; I personally believe due to its severe toxicity, **Comfrey is NOT a safe herb**.

STRAWBERRY

Fragaria vesca

Teas made from strawberry leaves are useful as a tonic for the control of diarrhea in children.

SORREL

Rumex acetosa

It is also called sourgrass; leaves and roots are used for cleaning blood and deworming; and the leaves are eaten as salads to prevent scurvy.

CROW FOOT

Geranium maculatum

It is a 1-2 foot erect plant with purple flowers; the leaves are deeply parted and toothed; flowering cycle is April-May. The dried roots and leaves are used as an astringent for the treatment of dysentery and internal hemorrhoids.

NOTE: Leaves and roots contain high tannins, a useful remedy for diarrhea and possibly an antibiotic effect.

RED CLOVER

Trifolium pretense

It is a very common weedy plant. The flowering tops boiled with added sugar is used as an antispasmodic for whooping cough. It is a good blood purifier and bitter tonic. It is considered useful in cancer treatment and a cure for hot flashes.

BALM OF GILEAD

Populus candicans

A favorite of Catfish which he called, Callum **Balma Gilea.** Flower buds boiled in olive oil are used as a salve for healing and soothing of joints as well as for dry cough and asthma.

HOREHOUND

Marrubium vulgare

It is useful in cough remedies, produces excessive sweating, relieves chronic sore throat, and asthma. Boil in a pint of water with 2 tablespoons of honey.

CHICORY

Cichorium intybus

It is a common weed of waste places and grows in every parking lot in West Virginia. It is also called Blue Soldiers. At full noon the flowers are open and stand erect and resemble a line of soldiers standing in for inspection. The root has medicinal value. It has been used as a coffee substitute. It is a mild laxative, increases urine flow, and useful to treat upset stomach. The leaves and flowers are edible and can be used in salads with other greens.

YELLOW DOCK

Curly dock Rumex crispus

The root has medicinal value. Hot tea is useful for superficial swelling and wounds, sores, and itchy skin conditions. It is also useful as a tonic, and may decrease diarrhea (due to high tannins).

YARROW

Achillea millefolium

The entire plant is useful. It is good for breaking a cold, used to break fever, and it also increases urine flow. It is an excellent douche for white discharge, and it can be used as an enema for hemorrhoids. The tea made from the flowers is good for stopping the bleeding of superficial wounds.

BLACK COHOSH

Cimicifuga racemes

Black Cohosh is a perennial herb that grows up to 6-8 ft tall. This plant is topped with spikes of white flowers. It is an effective, well established treatment of menopause symptoms, such as hot flashes, decreased libido, and depression. **Note:** Early colonial's used it for bronchitis, nervous disease, and rheumatism (tea made from the root). It also relieves menstrual cramps and spasms. It is a general herbal tonic not to be used in pregnancy.

DITTANY

Conila origanoides

It is seldom mentioned in European medicine, however early settlers were very familiar with it and used it against horseflies by sticking a bunch into the horses saddle. It was well known and used by early farmers as a tea concoction for colds and fevers, as well as nervous headaches. Mr. Catfish used tea for chest colds and mild feverish conditions.

WORM WOOD

Artemisia absinthium[2]

It is an old remedy for expelling worms and is also used for liver problems. A cloth soaked in hot tea made of the leaves is good for sprains and bruises. One teaspoonful of the leaves boiled in water is good to increase appetite. Wormwood was a popular bitter tonic ingredient of alcohol in the19th century. Due to its severe side effects of seizure, delirium, and hallucinations it has been banned.

WAHOO

Euonymus atropupureus

A medium sized tree with purple flowers. The bark of the tree has been used in Appalachia as a bitter tonic, laxative, expectorant and diuretic. It was quite popular in the early 1920's in West Virginia as a general tonic.

COMPASS PLANT- WILD LETTUCE

Lactuca scariola

According to Mr. Catfish, God had created the Milky Way and evening star to guide you at night and compass plants to guide your way during the day. The leaves of this plant twist and

---

[2] According to ancient writers, it was considered an antidote against mushroom and hemlock poisoning. Painter Van Gogh was addicted to wormwood in alcohol and some of his last paintings were painted in the vision of hallucination as a result of it.

turn facing the sun, and keeping one edge toward the sun--north and south, for that reason it is called a compass plant. The juice of the plant has a sedative effect and was given to babies to calm them down. It was also used as a treatment for sore throat, nervous tonic, and to increases urine and milk flow. **Note:** It belongs to the Aster family, reproduced by seeds, it has a milky juice highly lobed or prickly marginated leaves. The leaf tips point north and south. The leaves are vertical to better withstand the hot summer sun. The milky resin was used by Native American's as chewing gum. Some Indians believed lightening occurred more frequently where compass plant grew and would not camp there.

Wild lettuce is an ancestor of much garden lettuce. The stem and leaves are deeply cut and have sharp toothed margins. When the milky juice turns brown it resembles opium. It is used to treat insomnia, colic and diarrhea. Early leaves are edible, while older ones are quite bitter.

Look at this vigorous plant that lifts its head from the meadow see how its leaves are turned to the North. As true as the magnet. This is the compass-flower that the finger of God has planted.

Evangeline A tale of Acadie
Henry Wadsworth Longfellow

VERVAIN

Verbena hastate

Vervain is a perennial herb with angular stems and small lilac flowers. It is used as a bitter tonic, diuretic, for kidney and bladder complaints, and is also useful in colds and chest complaints, sore throat and asthma. **It contains iridous glycosides** (Verbenalins).

POKE BERRY

Phytolacea americana

This is a large herbaceous plant that has fleshy leaves, greenish white flowers and dark purple berries. The root is used medicinally, however the berries are poisonous. Young leaves are used early and if well prepared are edible. Older leaves are not as well prepared and could be harmful. It is a laxative and has a slight narcotic effect, as well as a slow acting emetic. Poke weed, can be boiled and eaten like asparagus or cooked like spinach, when boiled it can be applied to sores or one may **bath the head as a remedy for high blood pressure.** Poke weed contains steroid like ingredients and helps skin conditions such as psoriasis, acne, and fungal infections.

Note: Berries contain colored alkaloids **betacyanines** and was used in the past to color red wine. The plant contains lectins, saponins which explain its effect on arthritis, viral infections, diuresis, spermicidal, hypotension. **It does have toxic properties.**

SOLOMON SEAL

Polygonatum multi florum

Teas made from its roots are good for female complaints and it is also useful as a wash for poison ivy and external wounds. It is good for vomiting, freckles, and helps in healing wounds and broken bones.

ANGELICA

Angelica atropurpurea

This is a shrub 7-8 feet tall. The stem is purple colored with greenish white flowers. There are toothed leaflets at the tip of the leaf's stem. Though the roots of the plant have been used to treat bloating and stomach problems the seeds have also been used to prevent alcoholism. Mr. Catfish only used this herb for female troubles, mainly difficult menstrual periods because it helps in the improvement of menses. It is also used for rheumatic complaints of joints. A tea made from the roots or seeds help uterine contractions and improves libido in women. This tea also improves vision, hearing, and expulsion of afterbirth (placenta).

Because of its multiple benefits, Mr. Catfishh's opinion was favorable for its use in many female complaints. According to Mr.

Catfish, *Angelica* was used in epidemics to strengthen the heart, that is why the name 'Archangel'. Mr. Catfish uses ginger combined with angelica as a '**sex pepper up'.**

GOLDEN SEAL

Hydrastis canadensis

These perennial plants are 1-2 feet high. It has one stem with 2-5 lobed leaves, greenish white flowers, and the root is bright yellow. Tea made from the root is useful as an antibiotic, sore throat, diarrhea, and inflamed eyes. Mixed with grease, it is an excellent insect repellant.

HYSSOP

Hyssopus officinalis

Purge me with hyssop and I shall be clean,
Wash me and I shall be whiter than snow.
Psalms 51:7

Hyssop is known since biblical times. It is useful for stomach problems, asthma, and effective in cough and cold remedies. The tea is useful for treatment of intestinal worms.

QUEEN OF MEADOW

Eupatorium pupureum

It is also called Joe Pye Weed and Gravel root. It is a perennial, with a hollow stem growing 8-10 feet tall, 4-6 whole leaves, flowers are purple. Root and whole herb was used by Native Americans for breaking fevers. It also apparently was used extensively to treat typhus fever in the 19th century. It is a mild diuretic and increases urine flow, for that reason it was used for urinary infections and bladder stones. It is a general tonic. The instructions for use are as follows: Take 15 drops of tincture in water.

GERMAN CHAMOMILE

Matricaria recutita

A perennial herb, the leaves are pale green and the flower heads are yellow white and daisy like, apple scented. Teas made from flowers are a good tonic. It has a good sedative effect.

FRINGE TREE- OLDMAN'S BEARD

Chioanthus virginica

A small to medium tree, smooth oval leaves, with white ribbon like flowers in dense clusters. Tea made from inner bark is used as a tonic. Also helps urine flow, external wounds, cuts and bruises, and is useful in diarrhea and sore throat.

RABBIT TOBACCO-FUZZY GUSSY

(SWEET EVERLASTING)

Psuedognaphalium obtusifolium

It is a small herbaceous plant, narrow alternate leaves flowers whitish bloom (very tiny) plant is has a wool appearance and it grows in waste places in the late summer. It was used by Native Americans instead of tobacco for its mystic and spiritual powers. It has a sedative and diuretic effect and relieves mild pain. It has been used for bronchial irritation, cough, and asthma.

SASSAFRAS

Sassafras officinale

A small tree with **mitten shaped leaves.** There are three different types of leaves (triple, double, and single lobed). It has yellow flowers. The female and male species occur on separate trees. The peeled bark of the root is a good spring tonic to thin your blood and purify it. It is a tonic used for the stomach, and is also good for inflamed eyes. If chewed, the leaves are useful for a toothache. Sassafras tea is refreshing and if used as a general tonic, helps colic and other stomach ailments.

SAGE

Salvia officinalis

Why should a man die whilst sage grows in his garden.

Sage is useful in many conditions such as high fevers, bronchitis, palsy, nerves, flatulence, sore throat, and to stop milk flow from the breast milk. Sage is an ancient herb dedicated to the Greek god Zeus (Roman Jupiter) from *salvus* means **save.** It belongs to the mint family. Leaves are of medicinal value and have been considered a cure all, or a herb useful for all reasons. Boil a teaspoonful of leaves in 8 oz of water, and you may add honey, use it as a gargle for sore throat, or drink as a tea to help relieve hot flashes or night sweats.

Sage tea is good for wound care and helps in healing of sores. It also helps remove dandruff, treat headaches, and nervous excitement. Sage is not included in the BITTERS.

SLIPPERY ELM

(Red Elm, Indian Elm)

Ulmus rubra

It is a medium size tree, with a trunk dividing into widespread limbs; crown is broad and flat topped. It grows in moist rich soils. Flowers are stalk less, with opened leaves from February to May. Leaves are long, unequally toothed, with rough hair on both sides. The inner bark of the tree has medicinal value and has been an official drug of United States pharmacopoeia. The bark is collected in the spring. The wood has no commercial value. Strips of bark can be bent without breaking, and when moistened swells up.

It is a traditional herbal medicine used in Appalachia since the times of early settlers and Native Americans. It can be used as pudding and as nutritious food. It has soothing effects on wounds and stomach ailments (gastritis, colitis) and is useful in indigestion, labor pains, dysentery, bronchitis, cough, and hemorrhoids. It is also used in many over the counter cough tablets.

BONESET

Eupatorium perfoliatum

These perennial herbs grow 5-6 feet high with perfectly opposite leaves and joined together (which is why it is called 'bone'). The stem seems right in the middle of the leaves, with white flower clusters of flat heads. It grows in moist, swampy areas. It is one of the most important herbs in Appalachia. Tea made from its leaves acts as a laxative. It is used for fever, pneumonia, chest colds, and rheumatism. It is used to break bone fever or Dengue fever by using 2 tablespoonfuls of dry leaves in 8 oz of water. Drink with honey or brown sugar once or twice a day for pneumonia or Dengue fever.

HORSERADISH

Early Irish- Scottish settlers in Appalachia brought along the traditions of planting horseradish. The roots are mainly used in medicine and as a relish for roast beef sandwiches. The root was cut, grated, or rubbed on sore joints for rheumatism. Horseradish was also rubbed on the forehead for headache. It has a strong natural decongestant chemical **allyl isothiocyanate** which opens the sinus passages by inhalation of vapors. Therefore if the headache is due to clogged sinuses, it may be relieved by explanation of this folk remedy.

Note: Horseradish has been used in diet drinks. According to Mr. Catfish, this herb is under the effects of Mars. Its juices are effective for scurvy, scorbutic sores, bleeding gums, and jaundice.

INDIAN TOBACCO

Lobelia inflata

A branding herbaceous plant, usually 1-2 feet high with tiny white flowers. Seed pods are round bladder-like structures. The bottoms of the flowers are inflated. Indian tobacco is useful in asthma and epilepsy. The powdered leaves act like nicotine because it contains lobeline alkaloid.

ALUM ROOT- CROWFOOT, CRANESBILL

Geranium maculatum

It works as a powerful drying agent or astringent action used internally, for diarrhea and dysentery. Externally used as a douche or enemas, especially hemorrhoids. When mixed with equal parts of golden seal and boiled in water it is useful for mucus discharge from the bladder and intestine. It is helpful with nosebleeds, profuse menstruation, bleeding wounds, and chronic ulcers on the legs.

SUMACH BERRIES

Rhus glabra

A shrub or small tree, the leaves are 1-2 feet long with multiple leaflets. The fruit is bright red and velvety. It is very useful for the treatment of syphilis, gonorrhea, and fevers. Tea gargles are useful for sore throats, mouth sores, and fevers.

MULLEIN

Verbascum thapsus

Grows in dry fields, it is biennial, the first year the leaves grow and the second year it begins flowering; has long flannel teal leaves. The flowering stalk reaches 6-7 feet high with yellow flowers. Teas made from the flowers are good for many respiratory complaints such as bronchitis and cough. It also promotes urine flow (diuretic). The root burned and inhaled is good for asthma. When boiled the leaves are good to wrap around sprains and bruised limbs. When boiled in olive oil the flowers can be used as an earache medicine.

MILKWEED

Asclepias syriaca

A perennial herb which grows to 5-6 feet tall, broad oval leaves with a fuzzy under surface, with purple and white flowers in the head. The roots are collected in the fall. It improves the flow of urine. It is an effective treatment for poison ivy by using its white milky secretions, which neutralizes poison ivy (dermatitis) skin lesion. Mr. Catfish recommends two plants, Solomon Seal and Hemp, for the treatment of poison ivy dermatitis as well as the milky sap is useful for the treatment of warts.

BUTTERNUT

Juglans cinerea

This is a white walnut, blooming June through August, the fruit is long and pointed about 1 ½ inches, and is covered with a hairy husk. The inner bark is a very useful laxative with smooth actions. Mr. Catfish used it to treat bleeding gums.

DOCK

There are two types; narrow leaved curly dock (*rumex crispus* L.) and broad leaf dock (sour dock). They are usually found on the river banks or waste places. Young leaves are excellent for green salads or combined with spinach. The medicinal values of curly dock range from cleaning the liver, to crushing the leaves for treatment of skin boils, or using the juice for ringworms (especially in vinegar extract) and hives. The fresh root is used as a laxative and to cleanse the liver.

BLACK WALNUT

Juglans nigra

Mr. Catfish used black walnut in his bitter tonic for its excellent astringent taste and color. It has been an ingredient in various herbal concoctions since early medieval times. It is one of the secret inert ingredients which imparts certain color and taste, which is hard to obtain by any other means. Hair washed with tea made from green walnuts gives an excellent black shiny appearance. Tea made from peeled green outer layers is useful for intestinal worms, treatment of skin ulcers wounds, and nail fungus infections.

BLACKBERRY

Rubus villosus

Roots and leaves are excellent for intestinal flux, diarrhea of any kind, internal bleeding, and vomiting. Medicinal effects are due to strong astringent effect. It can be used as a tea, made from roots, and a fruit jelly or syrup, which is useful for diarrhea. Blackberry juice or jellies are important preserves both as a food source and medicinal value for treatment of diarrhea. **Note:** An important treatment in Appalachia for nausea, vomiting, and diarrhea: take blackberry tea every 2 hours until resolved.

BLUE COHOSH

Caulophyllum thalictroides

Blue cohosh is a perennial plant with greenish yellow flowers, and blue berries in the late summer. It is used as a stimulant, it increases menstrual flow, and is used to treat hiccups. Mr. Catfish avoided use the use of this plant because of the often misuse in abortions. It was used effectively to facilitate delivery of a child by using it as a tea 2-3 weeks before childbirth because it helps contractions of the uterus.

ANISE

Ozmorrhiza longistyles

Anise is sometimes called, 'sweet cicely'. Anise grows in low lying moist lands. It is useful in gas pains (flatulence). It helps alleviate cough symptoms and is a good cold remedy.

MAYAPPLE

Podophyllum peltatum

It is native plant that occurs in colonies. It has dark brown roots and is very fibrous. The leaves are large palmate heart shaped single lemon whit flower fruit nature in late summa. It is an excellent laxative (strong) emetic.

INDIAN HEMP

Apocynum cannabinum

It is about 3 feet high and has a milky white juice. It acts as a diuretic and diaphoretic. It is also useful for local poison ivy dermatitis.

THYME

Thymus vulgaris

Are you going to Scarborough Fair,
parsley, sage, rosemary and thyme.
Remember me to one who lives there
She once was a true love of mine.

It is a small herbaceous plant with numerous erect stems, less than one foot high, leaves are long ovate, flowers are bluish purple and small, arranged in whorled spikes. It is useful for throat and bronchial irritation, and whooping cough. It is used to ease headaches and nervousness. It was used in the past to cure hangovers, to kill intestinal parasites, disinfect wounds, and to treat urinary tract infections.

In the middle ages, legend says that sleeping on thyme pillows will get rid of melancholy and help one be courageous. **Note:** Thyme was given to sheep and goats to increase milk production, according to Mr. Catfish. Thyme is an herb of Venus, safe and speedy delivery to women in birth ensures a remedy for nightmares. Used by Egyptians in embalming. The active ingredient in Thyme is an antiseptic and is useful in mouth wash and as tooth paste.

CHAMOMILE

Anthemis nobilis

It is a good bitter tonic; it helps spasmodic conditions, menstrual flow, regulate menses, good eye wash, poultice for sprains, and swelling.

BLOOD ROOT

Sanguinaria canadensis

The natives call it red pucoon any coloring

It was used for sore throat and the treatment of piles, or to induce vomiting. **Note:** Plant is toxic and has very limited use in tooth paste industry.

CATNIP

Nepata cataria[3]

A perennial herb with hairy leaves and small pink blue flowers arranged in round clusters. Some of the medicinal uses of the flowers and leaves are colic, spasms, and gas in children. It is helpful for migraine headaches. Marshmallow root mixed with catnip is an excellent remedy for children.

---

3 The calming effect is due to nepetalactone , a compound belonging to iridous similar to valerian which has pheromone activity with a cat's courtship behavior, it is used in cat toys to have a playful effect. It is a good insect repellent.

AMERICAN DITTANY

Cunila mariana

American dittany is a small indigenous herb, found in dry shady hills; blooming in June and July and having a fragrant odor. Its infusion helps sweating and the treatment of mild fever. It promotes suppressed menstruation, relives flatulence, and colic. It is closely related to mint and penny royal in medicinal properties.

HOPS[4]

Humulus lupulus

The flowers of hops have medicinal properties. It is useful for anxiety disorders, is valuable for alcohol withdraws, and is a good toothache remedy. It increases the flow of urine and is a good nerve tonic. Hops can be stuffed in pillows for a good nights sleep.

---

[4] Hops are ripe catkin of a hop, added to malt liquor (beer) it provides a bitter taste to beer as opposed to fruity taste without hops, it stabilizes and preserves beer thus allowing it to both keep and travel. The first mention of it is in 10 th century in the regions of Europe predominantly beer drinking.

SELF HEAL

Prunella vulgaris

He that hath self heal needs no other physician.

Self heal is a small low plant, with round pointed leaves like and it blooms in May. The entire plant is useful for various ailments. It helps to stop bleeding. It is also useful for epilepsy. According to Mr. Catfish it is the herb of Venus. This is a special herb for inward and outward wounds. It is good for both mouth ulcers and headaches. According to Gerard, Bugle and Self Heal, are two excellent herbs for the treatment of wounds.

MEDICINE WAYS

OF THE

SIMPLE FOLKS

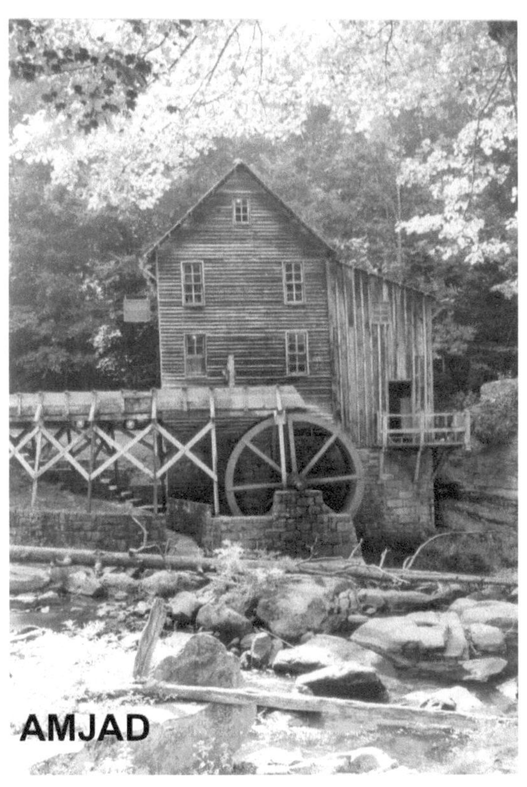

HERBAL REMEDIES OF CATFISH

TREATMENT OF POISON IVY

Catfish recommended the following herbs:

1. White milk juice of milkweed
2. Hemp juice
3. Wild lettuce

DIARRHEA

Flux

Mr. Catfish recommended first choice blackberry root tea or crow's foot (Geranium) along with horehound which decreases spasms of the bowel. Blackberry root tea is effective in treatment of dysentery or blood flux. He also suggested three glasses of lemonade in summer and one glass of it in the winter. A cup of sassafras in the summer time, use of celery, beets and green beans help blood flux. He suggested lemonade and sassafras tea help prevent blood flux.

GENERAL TONICS

Mr. Catfish recommended the use of dill pickles, olives, and olive oil with salads. To promote excellent health he suggests Ginseng tea and tea made of Queen of Meadows (flowers).

CURE FOR GALLSTONES

Mr. Catfish suggested drinking 8 oz of water with one teaspoonful of baking soda taken twice a day for one week, then once at night for two weeks.

FOOD POISONING

The Appalachian Two Way Virus (diarrhea and vomiting). Mix ½ teaspoonful of nutmeg powder in one ½ pint of milk, take several doses until symptoms have stopped.

ANISEED

Aniseed is useful for headaches (Migraine), cold and cough.

YEAST INFECTION

Sage tea is useful to take also bathe the affected part.

LAXATIVE

Mr. Catfish recommended

1. **Head of Lettuce**

3 leaves a day will cure constipation in a lot of people.

(Comments: this is a very inexpensive high fiber diet which has sound medical advice and it is very possible to follow, except in the elderly and people who have difficulty chewing due to poor dental statues).

2. **Applebutter or Apple sauce**

2 tablespoons every day.

3. **Summac Berries**

4. **Solomon Seal or a berry,** which is a strong laxative and has old tradition for its use.

5. **Mayapple root** is a very strong laxative.

CURSE OF TOMATO FAMILY

DIETARY ADVICE

According to Mr. Catfish avoid following foods:

Eggplant

Tomatoes

Potatoes Instant coffee (possible pancreatic cancer)

Web footed fowls (such as ducks)

Round hoofed animals (horse)

No birth control pills (cancer, blood clots, strokes, migraine)

Mr. Catfish had strong feelings against tomatoes, which he attributed to causing cancers in the Western World. According to Mr. Catfish, both tomatoes and potatoes belong to the Night shade family where well known poisonous plants occur. **Note:** This belief goes back to earlier European views of poisonous tomatoes.

Mr. Catfish may have a solid scientific point of view due to the many side effects of these food products which has became part of everyday life. He was not in favor of other food items which are products of the modern day general food industry and believed all of these have several underlying health problem, such as:

Carbonated Drinks (obesity, dyspepsia, irritable bowel syndrome)

Salt (high blood pressure arteriosclerosis)

Artificial Sweeteners (headache, migraine, chronic fatigue)

Fish without Scales (these are bottom of stream scavengers and have high level of toxins such as mercury, PCB, and other man made disasters, which interfere with the optimum pH (homeostasis pH of 7.4 which is slightly alkaline) of human organs. As the body turns acidic, slight major malfunctions of various body organs may begin. We often eat foods which have lots of acid and our bodies try to dispose of this acid. By taking a small quantity of baking soda you are helping your body tremendously, because the kidneys, liver, and lungs are working hard to conserve alkali and dispose acid, so they can maintain the ideal pH (homeostasis).

BRIEF REVIEW

Avoid the following foods:

Pork

Cabbage

Eggplant

Tomatoes

Oranges

Sugar

Take ½ teaspoons of baking soda in 8 oz of water daily to keep kidneys from being gummed up.

Catfish also recommends the following herbs to help one begin menses:

Coltfoot

Verbain

Ginger Tea is a good remedy to start the menstrual cycle (emenogoque). Irregular menstrual periods are a cause of many diseases of women, such as PMS, headaches, abdominal cramps, and pelvic pain. This is a simple remedy that is not often utilized.

SULPHUR THERAPY

For the use of any illnesses such as diabetes, multiple sclerosis, or Parkinson's (neurological disorders) disease:

¼ teaspoons of Epsom salt

¼ teaspoons of Cream of Tartar

¼ teaspoons of sulphur

HUMAN PHYSIOLOGY

A Short Cut

(Approach by Mr. Catfish)

Most of the above mentioned food products such as artificial sweeteners and beverages can be digested by the stomach, but they later "gum up" the kidney, in so leading to formation of a goiter, tumors, heart attack, gall stones, kidney stones, diabetes, and hardening of the arteries. Good healthy food will not 'gum up' the kidney, this way the kidneys will be able to get rid of what the body does not need.

Note: DARWIN'S MEDICINE in a nut shell, is the concept of medicine looked through evolution of basic physiological principles, for example, fever is a useful response because it triggers the body to fight infection (or other causes). Excessive attempts to lower the fever are not helping the body and prolong the infection such as flu symptoms, etc. Nausea and vomiting during pregnancy is "protective" so the mother will avoid harmful foods which can cause problems to the fetus. It is known that women who have severe nausea and vomiting during pregnancy that their newborn will have less health problems than those who do not. Human teeth are modeled as grinder of grains and bean and not canine flesh eating animals, therefore excess meat eating is unphysiologic according to tenets of Darwin's medicine.

The human body was built and modified through evolutionary processes of a mixed diet of grains, vegetables, lentils, and so is the digestive system and pancreas. Excessive use of refined food products such as sugars, carbonated drinks, and excessive salt are all unphysiologic according to Darwin's medicine.

Catfish recommends

INSOMNIA	lobelia
IMPOTENCE	baking soda
FRECKLES	tansy

HOW TO MAKE BITTERS

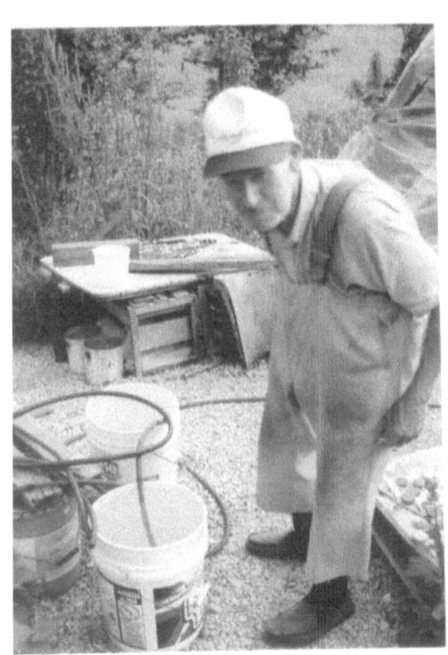

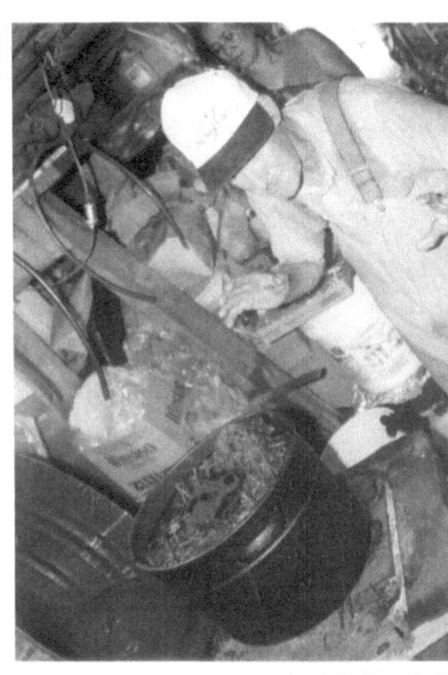

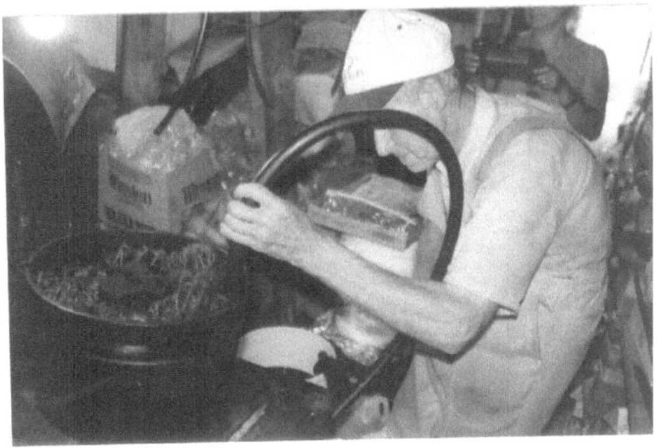

SONG OF CATFISH'S BITTERS

-Hassan Amjad, 2003

Wahoo,

Boil them fast, put spikenard in the charmed pot

Hyssop and Hops and what ever grows in the back lot

No eye of newt no toes of frogs

But golden seal , sassafras dug fresh from the Boggs.

No wool of a bat, no lizard leg in that what

boils and bubbles

Yarrow, but not tomorrow take you women with troubles

No adder's fork and blind worm's sting

Nature's gift of herb me and then sing

What round about cauldron goes

Roots and flowers, spring water I throw

Keep going till the moon's eclipse

Or you hear catfish's bitters from every lips.

Macbeth
Shakespeare
with apologies

Sassafras, Ginseng round me stacked
With Dittany, Lobelia together hurled
Slippery Elm, Great Solomon Seal,
Black Cohosh stuffed and packed
Such is my world! And what a world

Hassan Amjad
(With apology to **FAUST**)

BITTER TONICS

Mr. Catfish was renowned for his bitter tonics, (a detailed account is subject of a separate volume) a brief summary below is provided. He apparently learned the use of these combinations from Native American Indians. The following 15 herbal formulas were commonly used:

Ginseng	Golden Seal
Spikenard	Blood Root
Joe Pye Weed	Wild Cherry
Comfrey	Mayapple
Black Cohosh	Solomon Seal
Sassafras	Blue Lobelia
	Slippery Elm
	Yarrow

Weigh one ounce of the herbs dried leaves, (2 oz if not dried) in 2 ½ gallon of water and boil down to 1 gallon and a quart of water. **Strain Well.** Mr. Catfish used cotton socks as a filtering device and they worked wonderfully. Keep this tea refrigerated or in a dark, dry, and cool place. To sweeten this tea use wildflower honey, one pint of honey to 2 pints of water, mix and refrigerate. Mr. Catfish always uses spring water and no aluminum pots!

For cancer use the following herbs:

Burdock root

Yellow Dock root

Pipsissewa

Peppermint

Red Clover blossom

For menopause

Yarrow and Pipsissewa

For 'sex up'

Ginseng

Spikenard

Joe Pye Weed

For blood purifier

Sassafras

Golden Seal

Blood root

Wild Cherry

For laxative

Mayapple

Solomon Seal

HOW TO USE BITTERS

For general tonic: 2 tablespoonful 3 times a day before meal. For cancer Bitter: 3 tablespoonful 3 times a day

ASTROLOGY

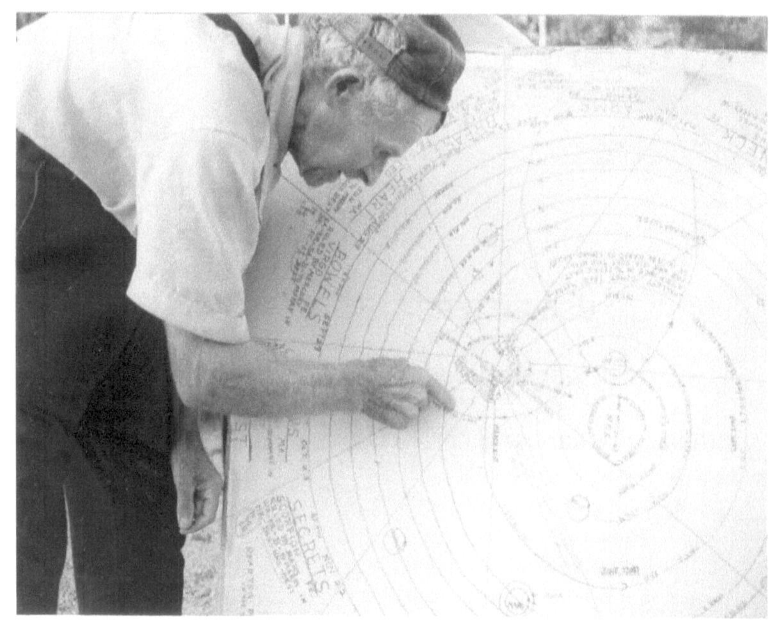

A DOCTOR OF MEDICINE

With us there was Doctour of Physik

for being grounded in astronomye.

He watched his patients favorable star

and by his Natural Magic knew what are

the cause of every malady you'd got

the cause knowne, send him drogges and his

lecturaries.

Prologue to The Canterbury Tales
Geoffrey Chaucer
(1340-1400)

When the planets in evil mixture to disorder wander

What plagues and what portents.

Troilus and Cressida
I, iii, 94
Shakespeare

ASTROLOGY

Mr. Catfish was a man of religion and a devoted Christian, his belief in Astrology here is no conflict. According to him, God created the heaven and stars and it is not against the best Christians to guide your behavior by the stars.[5] According to Mr. Catfish, people get diseases in cycles every 28 days. Because when each person's astrology (zodiac) signs come up, that person is susceptible for two days.

One of the **principles of astrology** is the assignment of Zodiac signs and celestial planets to body parts and their diseases under the influence of planetary changes.

SATURN	Teeth, spleen, bones
JUPITER	Liver- Lungs, veins
MARS	Gall bladder
VENUS	Sexual organs, kidney, breast
MERCURY	Brain, locomotive power
SUN	Heart, eyes, sight
MOON	Stomach, bowels, bladder

[5] Plants should be collected with position of the planets in the heaven; Herbs which benefit male should be collected in Sagittarius and Aquarius or at Leo herb to benefit the female should be gathered under the female sign of Virgo or Taurus or Cancer.

ZODIAC SIGNS

ARIES	Anything above the neck, head
TAURUS	Neck
GEMINI	Hands, shoulders
CANCER	Breast, lung, liver
LEO	Heart
LIBRA	Kidney bladder
SCORPIO	Sexual organs
SAGITARIUS	Hips, coccyx
CAPRICORN	Knee, hamstring
AGUARIUS	Leg
PISCES	Feet, ankles
SUN	Causes disease of heart, brain
MOON	Drunkenness, cold, stomach ache
SATURN	Depression, melancholy, madness
JUPITER	Liver, vein disease, fever pleurisy
MARS	Anger, violent, passion, fever
VENUS	Love, genitourinary disease
MERCURY	Vertigo, brain diseases

Explanation of the Zodiac signs can be considered as a medicine specialist in modern sense.

SATURN	Psychiatric diseases
MARS	Infectious disease, epidemiology
MOON	Rheumatologist
VENUS	Gynecologist
MERCURY	Sports medicine

Opposite forces

Venus	vs.	Mars
Mercury	vs.	Jupiter
Saturn	vs.	Light (sun/moon)

Willow tree (*Salix* sp.) belongs to the moon since ancient times. The willow was sacred and grown around the temples of the Moon Goddess (Hecate, Hera, Persephone, and Circe). The Moon rules the water element, therefore trees favor water and grow around the streams and rivers. So according to Medieval herbalists, fevers or painful swellings of joints was like inside fir burning (inflammation). So fire could be extinguished by lunar herbs, because of its affinity for water. This is why the Willow tree had a reputation to treat fevers and inflammatory joints. Modern aspirin came from the bark of Salicylic acid[6], came from the bark of a willow.

God almighty has imprinted on plants, flowers, leaves, very signature of their virtues and their intrinsic value. So walnut is a perfect brain food (because appearance of walnut is like a brain.) Pomegranate with bright red seeds is good for the teeth.

---

6 Salicyclic acid derived from salix (willow tree) word Sal derives old celtic word which means near water Sal water, lis near. Aspirin came from related species spirea bush by addy just later.

LOOK YE

APHORISMS OF CATFISH

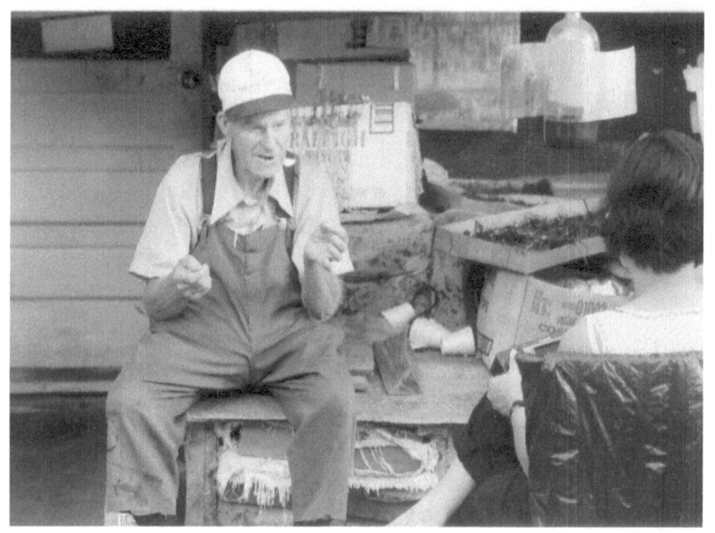

APHORISMS

They say an old man is twice A child

Hamlet II, ii, 39

Shakespeare

- I was a poor boy most of my life without education and found my way in the dark to where I am now
- God said to be ye temperate in all things
- It is good to know that things half done is never done still it is good to know that.
- Physics without reason is like pudding without fat

Culpepper

- Sweet Anise good remedy for bronchial complaints
- Indian Hemp is useful for stomach problems
- Yellow root taken regularly help keeps you in good health
- For vision problems us the following herbs:

  Spikenard

  Ginseng

  Angelica

- Mayapple root if chewed at night gives a perfect bowel movement in the morning
- Angelica is a good sex pepper upper especially when used with ginseng.

- For scabies combine the following :

Sulfur and Camphor

Sassafras King

Mr. Catfish spent years digging and preparing sassafras roots and was known as the sassafras king. He used the early spring flowers of sassafras as a tea or made it into jelly syrup. During the fall, burning sassafras leaves, got rid of molds, bugs, and moths.

Poison Ivy

Black Staining sap from the plants are poisonous, their antidote in milky white sap producing plants, such examples as poison ivy can be successfully treated with white sap of milk weed and hemp plant.

To start menstrual periods

He recommends the following:

1. Vervain (verbena officinalis)
2. Coltfoot
3. Ginger

This helps with increase the menstrual flow, and useful in combination with boneset and willow bark for treatment of fevers.

Bitter Stimulant

Ginseng

Angelica

Golden seal

Spikenard

Black cohosh

Slippery elm

Laxative

- Butternut
- Mayapple

Virginia Snakeroot

- For scarlet fever

Spikenard

- To improve vision or eyesight

Boneset

- For flu and pneumonia. Boil the leaves for 10 minutes one dose is enough

Queen of Meadow

- Cold
- Flu (boil the root for 10 minutes)

Chest Nut

- Good for whooping cough

Golden seal

- Gargles for sore throat, stomach ulcers

Author's Note:

Golden seal work as an antibiotic and is known since the early 19th century to possibly eradicate *H. pylori* causes of ulcers or gastritis. It is also an effective treatment for traveler's diarrhea.

- **Queen of Meadows** and Burdock: as treatment of cancer with bitters
- If you want to stay healthy avoid ketchup, tomato.
- **Crow's foot** (Geranium): for treatment of diarrhea
- **Black cohosh:** a good kidney medicine
- **Alum Root:** stops bleeding internally
- **Slippery Elm:** chew inner bark, slowly, good for stomach ulcers
- **Lobelia:** for use in insomnia and **impotence:** baking soda plus 1 teaspoon in a glass of water every night
- **Sex up Improvement** ginseng and ginger
- **Freckles** butter milk

NO TOMATOES

Mr. Catfish carried medieval belief that tomatoes are the cause of cancer because perhaps tomatoes are part of the night shade family and are poisonous (it is true that the leaves can be poisonous). In the 18th century, its Latin name reflected that belief 'Lycopersicon esculentum' or 'edible wolf's peach'. When the cause of polio was unknown, some people thought the paralysis was caused by eating tomatoes.

Tomatoes were initially used as an ornament due to superstition! Tomatoes are naturally found in the Andes and later became domesticated in Mexico. The original tomatoes were yellow (that's why they were called apples of gold). 'Pomodoro', which was misunderstood by the French as 'Pom d' Amore' or apple of love, was a symbol of an aphrodisiac. Many of the plants of the night shade family (Bella don) are poisonous so it is superstition with the eggplant.

MISCELLANEOUS

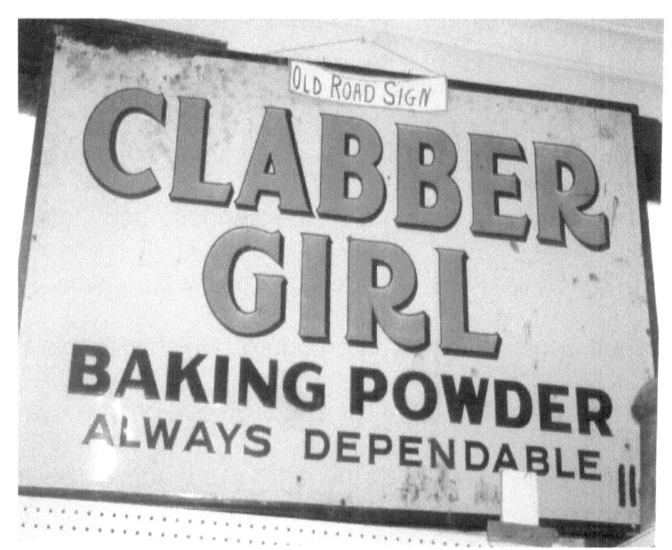

MR. CATFISH AND BAKING SODA

Mr. Catfish was very fond of using baking soda for many illnesses. His favorite uses were the treatment of diabetes, arthritis, and sex up remedies.

Special Note:

In early 1860, James Church operated a spice and mustard business, known as vulcan spice mills (according to Roman mythology Vulcan is the god of fire and blacksmiths. Shown fashioning arms etc for other gods he is shown arm of Vulcan, holding a hammer to hit anvil Arm & Hammer[7] trademark was used for packages of baking soda later became company logo.

BAKING SODA

The natural sources of soda are minerals of native soda, such as matron (in Egypt, Hungary and South America's it is called Trona in Egypt). Impure soda is derived from ashes of plants growing on the surface or bordering the sea and is called Barilla/kelp especially, of the genera, *Salsola*. In ancient times, *Salicornia* and *Chenopodiam* were cultivated (in Spain and Sicily) for yielding soda. When ripe, they were cut down, dried, and burnt so the ashes formed a hard fused mass.

---

[7] Arm & Hammer, the symbol was used in 1860, by James Church, founder of mustard business Vulcan Spice Mills. Vulcan, in Roman mythology, was the god of fire and was skilled in making arms for gods and heroes. The Arm & Hammer represented the arm of the god Vulcan, and this trade mark was later used on baking soda packages, which also become the trade mark for (Church & Dwight Co. Inc.). Manufacture of (bicarbonate of soda) baking soda started in US in 1846, cow brand was, because sour cow's milk was used in baking.

Spanish barilla contains 25% of sodium bicarbonate. Before the artificial production of Soda, these were the source of soda, it was mainly used for manufacturing of soaps in Paris, and its industrial use became available in1784, by Le Blane and Dize in England.

Baking Soda was used in conditions of increased acidity of the stomach, treatment of dyspepsia, gout, arthritis, as well as skin conditions when used as an external remedy.

HONEY BEES AND MR. CATFISH

Mr. Catfish knew the language of the honey bees. Their swarming and nesting psychology responds to certain metallic noises and vibrations, as well as changing their flight patterns. Catfish avidly collected wild honey and had excellent skills in gathering large quantities each year. Finding a bee tree is an old Appalachian tradition that requires some experience. Early settlers brought honey bees from Europe. The honey bees took to the woodlands of America including Appalachia. Wild honey dispending upon the source has certain favor and color. It is well know that bees favor yellow poplar trees and it gives a dark honey, while honey from black locusts has a lighter color. Other common plants are red maple, goldenrod, white clove and sour would.

Using traditional bee smokers, rags are burned in a metal portion and air bagged, creating cloud of rising smoke making honey bees move leaving the pot of their treasure. During one summer, one of Mr.

Catfish's neighbors was rude and cantankerous. Catfish rode by in his bicycle with the metal bell ringing and loudly! There followed swarms of honey bees leaving his neighbors collection. One medieval writings of Mattioli commentaries, (Lyon 1597) mentions how metal sound produce can redirect swarms of honey bees.

MOVEMENT OF PLANTS

Mr. Catfish was an astute observer of nature, whether it was a compass plant pointing north and south or a twining plant he was eager to show to visitors. According to him most of twining plants grow clockwise like morning glory.

REFERENCES

1. Greed Ted, Bennett Allen Catfish, The works and ways of a herb doctor Goldenseal page 46-51 vol3, No.3, 1977

2. Putnam Democrat Vol 129: No. 18 March 12, 1998 Aren Man is herbal Medicine expert

3. Staff reporter Carley McCullogh Catfish dictated Notes on astrology only summary is included

4. Herald dispatch by David Peyton May 22, 1992

5. Charleston Gazette-Mail Sunday. Life, taking control of images from the mountains, Marry

6. Wade Burnside 16 February 1997

7. Mason County Herbalist, when Los Angles Public libraries called a real American character full of malarkey, old wives tales and tall tales

8. Putnam Democrat March 12, 1998 Area man is herbal medicine expert Carley McCullough

9. Johnny Carson and David Letterman Pm Magazine Public television 1981 he was officially named American Best herbal healer

10. Catfish Clarence Grey feeds his body with herbs and Twinkies and his soul with the bible Herald Dispatch. October 11, 1979

11. **America's Best 100** Luouso and Paul Sterling Publishing Emperor NY NY 1980

12. **Newspaper clipping** Herald dispatch. May 8 1975 Mountain median man supplies many curls.

13. **Los Angeles Times** June 15, 1975 Mountain medicine man has cure for all ills.

14. **Monroe Evening New Midigam** June 30, 1975 Dash of sassafras bit of bark, Everything cancer to freckles.

15. **Los Angeles Time** June 15, 1975 Mountain medicine man, Has a cure for all ills calls his basement as goundhog hole

16. He has appearance John Carson and Letterman TOS has & BBC program 1986 A Doctor's Deton in America

EPILOGUE

A FAIR FACE WILL WHITHER

A GOOD HEART IS THE SUN

AND MOON

-KING HENRY

SHAKESPEARE

WHO WAS CATFISH AND HIS LEGACY?

A genius? A medieval tinkered? Encapsulated in a time frame of the 20th century. His modest living can remind one of the great English puritan preachers, John Bunyan. He had no telephone or other modern amenities of life, and he lived in a one room house next to a cemetery. He did not drink or smoke and he had a simple life, living on food and plants grown in his backyard, and on natural spring water. He was visited daily by large, diverse crowds seeking his advice. In my estimation he had more visitors than most modern physicians ever can dream of.

He was a pure naturalist, while we may not agree on Victorian views of sex. This subject was important to him as an herbalist, not being bashful about it because his opinion was sought so often. Mr. Catfish attended church three times a week and often quoted scripture from the Bible. He avoided soft drinks, commercial foods, and artificial preservatives.

Mr. Catfish was not a Faith Healer or a Shaman. Sometimes anthropologists want to label such an attempt to cast these people in a set frame of mind. He had no secrets and he advised people actively. He was devoid of showmanship, despite a celebrity status. He did not exploit anyone for personal gains. In my opinion he was a pure herbalist, one of a kind whose main concern was to help those who needed him.

I know where catfish rest

I know a bank

Where the wild Thyme blows

Where oxlips and nodding violet grows

Quite over canopied with luscious woodbine

With sweet musk- roses and with eglantine

-A midsummer Nigh't Dream
Shakespeare

www.ingramcontent.com/pod-product-compliance
Ingram Content Group UK Ltd.
Pitfield, Milton Keynes, MK11 3LW, UK
UKHW041920190726
13854UKWH00003B/1341

9 781411 662797